Life Inside My Head

Personal Journey of Life After an Acquired Brain Injury

Jordan Murrell

ISBN: 978-1-947247-08-6
Life Inside My Head
Copyright © by Jordan Murrell

For permission requests, write to the publisher at the address below.

Yorkshire Publishing
3207 South Norwood Avenue
Tulsa, Oklahoma 74135
www.YorkshirePublishing.com
918.394.2665

Thoughts

Imagine going to sleep one day, just to wake up the next and discover you have no memories. Imagine a chapter in your life that you can't get past, because of a previous conflict in it. Imagine living in a world full of dead ends and obstacles. Imagine a world where no one understands you, or the things you've been through. Imagine if you could wish all of your problems away, then would everything be okay?

Would you be satisfied with the outcome, or would you want more? If you could make one wish would it be greedy and selfish, or would it benefit life and the people in it? Imagine if it was like this, would you do what's right, or stay tight and look out for you? If I could make one wish it would not only appeal to me, but to everyone living within the world…If I had a magical lamp and rubbed it twice,

A Genie would appear and grant three wishes.
I could then wish all these things into existence
And watch them come true,
Or I could wish on a shooting star and wait a day or two,
Then all of my dreams would come true.
Wouldn't that be nice if only it were true,
Even so one or three wishes wouldn't do.
If only the fairytale was true,

My dreams would become reality and happiness would no longer seem temporary, or impossible….

It would then become a state of mind, and not one of being. Life would become easier and the world would be a better place, but unfortunately life doesn't work that way.

Genies aren't real and wishes are not instantly granted by a shooting star, but that doesn't mean that wishes and dreams can't come true. It just means that we have to work our hardest to achieve them. Life isn't supposed to be easy, if it was it wouldn't be worth living. Life is meant to be experienced, so that we can learn from our mistakes and better ourselves from them.

It's our experiences in life that make us who we are. It's what we do today that changes our future tomorrows; and it's the choices we make that send us down the pathway to our destiny. Life is given to us for one reason, and that reason is to live. Therefore, each day that comes to us brings with it purpose. This purpose is the reason why we were created and brought into existence.

The very fact we're still alive means this purpose hasn't been fulfilled. It can also mean there's another piece to the puzzle we have yet to find, but life shouldn't just be about achieving that purpose. Life should be enjoyed; therefore, each day lived is a gift, but not every day experienced is a joyous occasion. Many times we experience difficulties in our daily lives, which cause unhappiness.

These random occurrences can happen at any time, and can't always be avoided. Whenever these things take place, happiness seems so frail and many times we find ourselves angry, sad, frightened or confused. I know all too well about the stress these kinds of situations can cause. We're human and we can only handle so much, but what sets us apart is how we deal with those problems, and I choose to write.

If only I had a pencil and paper everywhere I went. Would I see a change in the world then? Would life truly improve, or would the world revolve around me wherever I moved. No one has the answer.

Many questions fill my head, such as why it happened and why I'm still here? Do I have a greater purpose in life, if so, what is it? Can somebody tell me? Will someone give me a hint or tell me why? However, no one has the answer.

Only I can find that answer, because this is my life; this is my journey. This is life inside my head, but no matter my struggles or battles in life I will not give up. I will do my best at being all that I can be in this second chance at life, and that's a promise I'll never break. So every day that I awake I remember this promise I made and throughout the day I know everything will be okay. I will not give up, I will find my way.

The good Lord will guide me everyday, as long as I continue moving forward, my joy will never go away. I will believe in Him and trust His word every step of the way. He's blessed me to come this far, I won't disappoint Him. I will continue moving forward, my journey isn't over. I will work my hardest at being the best I can be every day.

My happiness will not give out; the Devil can't take my joy away. I will never give in to evil, or the weak. I will stand strong every day of the week, but is standing strong enough, because this world is rough, and no matter where I go conflict is waiting at the front door. Every day since, I've been made fun of, or mistreated. I'm pushed to my limits daily, just so others can humor themselves, or see my frustration.

Many times I've asked myself why these things happen, am I really the problem. Well the answer to that question is no, I'm not the problem; they are, but it still hurts to know the people I once called friends would treat me this way. It's times like these that strengthen my sorrow, to know they're people out there waiting to make their next move on me for no reason at all.

It could be today or tomorrow I don't know when it will take place. Nor do I know the time or date, but neither will I wait to find out. At times I feel like nobody cares, that no one's aware of how I feel about the things that take place in my life. Sometimes I listen to what's being said and other times I try to block it out.

"You don't pay attention."

"You don't listen, and you move too slowly."

These things were said daily, to make me feel low.

My disabilities were used against me in order for those around me to feel prideful of themselves, and many times I didn't know who to turn to, or where to go for help. Sometimes I even became so angry and frustrated, that I couldn't help but weep. This went on many times as I found myself in the same situation, but through time I learned how to cope. I will never believe in the negative things someone has to say about me, instead I will overshadow the fact it could be true. The very minute I don't, it'll cause me to have low self-esteem, or a lack of self-confidence about myself.

It will then spread like a disease. It will swallow me whole and take over, slowly turning me into the gossip, or hurtful things that were said against me. Many times I tell myself you're not trying hard enough. Other times I throw in the towel and give up, but I've come to a point in life where I realize these things are just a phase; a phase that I must go through, in order to get to the next chapter in life.

Therefore, these things will soon come to an end, and I can only trust and believe that God put these things in place for a reason. Whatever that reason may be, I know it's just to prepare me for the road ahead.

"Life Inside My Head" isn't a psychological thing, or a crazy thing. It's just explaining to you how I think on a daily basis; the ups and downs in my life, how I feel about the world, and the things that take place in it. My likes and dislikes about my situation, and the things I continuously face, for you to fully understand. However, you would have to know what happened to me. The reason my life is the way it is. This is my story…

The Wreck

When I was eleven, I died from the result of a tragic car wreck. It was a hit and run, that caused my mother's car to run off the road. The person responsible stopped her car to watch it happen, and then she sped off. She did not care about the results of her actions, she did not care that my mother was injured in the process, and she didn't care that I was draining two pints of blood.

Once the car came to a halt, my mother asked if we were okay. She knew that my brother was. His screaming testified to that, but the one voice she didn't hear was mine. At that moment I was experiencing the most intense pain I'd ever felt. My neck was sprained, and my head was busted wide open.

Within a matter of seconds I would be dead. No one would hear my cries, or witness my screams for help, because at that very moment my attention wasn't focused on my pain. Right before the wreck took place I saw two bolts of light shoot past our car that vanished within the blink of an eye. What I saw defied belief and I couldn't believe my mind.

It was two bright figures, both a man and woman racing towards our demise. After seeing this, I became filled with shock. I didn't know if what I had seen was real, or if it was an illusion of the mind. I quickly became frightened when I noticed how fast our car was going. The scenery outside, was moving incredibly too fast. I thought, "I am losing my mind."

I had no idea what was going on, but my mother knew very well what was taking place. In fact, she was trying to prevent it from happening. Unfortunately the driver ramming us had too much force and agility to escape. That's when our car began to sprawl out of control, as it moved off the road.

That's also when my mother pulled the parking break lever; hoping that our car would come to a halt, but instead it continued down its path, eventually moving off the road, over an uneven surface; Causing it to flip over twice, hit two trees, a light pole, and land in a ditch wrapped around a tree.

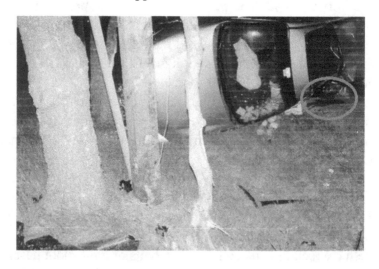

In the process smashing my head out the window, and causing me to hit many things. Then once we landed, the bright figures I saw earlier reappeared.

My eyes had not been deceived, they were angels. After appearing the male angel caught our car from the front, and the female the back left, also catching my head as it smashed outside my window. Then there came a point when her eyes and mine met. At that moment all was silent, I felt at peace and my pain didn't matter.

I felt secure, and I knew that I was going to be okay. Afterwards she softly stroked my face, gave a friendly smile, and waved goodbye. Then she slowly began to fade away from sight, along with her companion at the front of our car. Right after their departure, my mother began to call out for my brother and I. She hoped that we were both okay, but when she didn't hear me reply back, she knew I was hurt.

While I lay semiconscious, she began pulling on the hinges of her seatbelt. Once free from the belts safety lock, she fell into the ceiling, crawled out of her window, and progressed towards me. Once in sight, she saw my head gushing blood outside my window. After seeing this she began to weep, as she helplessly watched life drain away from me. The color in my face was growing pale, and the light in my eyes was becoming dim.

My life was slowly shifting out of balance, and my mother couldn't bear the thought. She then rolled over on her back, lifted both hands to my head, and tried her best to stop the blood from gushing out. The thought of death broke her heart and if she had anything to do with it she would save me; but what could she do? She was in no condition to move freely. All hope seemed lost, but my mother refused to give up on me.

She then cried out and said, "Don't you die on me Jordan Michael Murrell, don't give up!" I tried to respond back, but I could only gurgle blood instead. After using my last bit of strength to respond, I fainted in my mother's hand and had no idea of what took place next. Once she heard my response, she knew I was fighting to stay alive, and that gave her the strength to fight, too. My mother then began to scream for help.

For a while her voice was unheard, until three drivers from the dead traffic rushed towards the wrecked scene. Once my mother's screams were heard they all called 911 and offered their help. After their arrival my mother, whose cellphone had been lost somewhere in the wrecked vehicle, used one of theirs to contact my dad. Meanwhile another helping hand approached the scene.

It was a beautiful Caucasian female with long, curly, blond hair who came to us in a jogging suit. She was a stranger whom my mother never met before, but there was something about this woman that made my mother calm. There was something about her bright smile that took away the doubt, fear, and sorrow my mother was feeling. Once on the scene she helped my mother to her feet and sat her beside a tree, opposite of the car.

In this woman's presence my mother became speechless, and remained paralyzed. She just couldn't figure out what it was about this woman that had her acting in such a way. After helping my mother, the strange woman progressed towards my baby brother who was still very afraid and trapped inside the wrecked vehicle. Once in sight, she reached through the shattered window for his hand.

After grabbing her finger, she began to sooth him by using a soft voice. Once calmed, she pulled off the car door and took him out. Once outside, she unbuckled the guard around his chest, and belts in between his legs. Afterwards she lifted him into her arms, wiped his tears, and rocked him until he calmed down some more. She then returned him to my mother.

Not long after the kind lady's arrival, my dad sped onto the scene, leading behind him the paramedics, fire fighters and police. Once summoned everyone worked together to get me out the car, but what seemed to be a simple task, was not so easy after all. My left foot was stuck in the lower section of my door. Thereby, making it hard to pull me out, but after continuous effort, I was finally plunged outside of the wrecked vehicle.

Once removed from the car I was laid onto the ground, then in an attempt to stop blood loss, my dad took off his shirt and wrapped it tightly around my head. After that was done, the strange woman approached my body. She then lifted my feet, held them and began to pray, afterwards she moved towards my damaged head, where she knelt down, held it and prayed once more.

The prayer was not understood, no one knew what she was saying, because she was speaking in tongues the whole time. My mother was in the presence of an angel, and all she could do was stare. Once the angel was done praying, she turned towards my mother and revealed a smile. Then she told my mother that I was going to be okay, and that God was watching over us.

Afterwards the angel told my mother to call on Him, when you get weary, or begin to lack in faith. To remember that, "He loves you, and wants nothing but the best for you and your children." Afterwards she left and we never saw, or heard from her again, since then. At that time the police officers, called to the site, began collecting information from my mother and the three witnesses left on the scene.

Once answers to their questions were collected they found out what took place and the sequence of details in which it happened. They also found out that from the three witnesses, two men were neighbors and were headed in the same direction we were, and both knew the woman that ran us off the road, because she lived across the street from them. Once this information was obtained it was recorded. Then the police officers drove off to search for this woman.

Meanwhile the Care Flight Helicopter that was called earlier to come and get me flew in and landed. During this time the chief fire fighter was in the process of checking for a pulse. As he looked at my pale face he encountered no life and became frightened. At the time he could only think of his own children, and the thought of an innocent kid dying was too much to bear.

11

That's when he pulled out a stethoscope; put the tips in his ears and the diaphragm on my chest hoping to get a pulse from my heart or catch a glimpse of air moving through my lungs.

He found no signs of life and was unsuccessful on his first attempt. So he then squeezed three fingers around my wrist, placed two on the side of my neck, pleaded out to God and said, "Please let me get a pulse." After pleading faithfully he received two faint pulse beats. Then after letting out a sigh of relief, he helped roll me into the helicopter.

Once inside I was quickly strapped down, and we took off. After the helicopter took flight my mother was put in a wheel chair and loaded onto the ambulance with my brother, where his vitals were now being checked. Then the ambulance sped off in the same direction as the helicopter, towards Cook Children's Hospital.

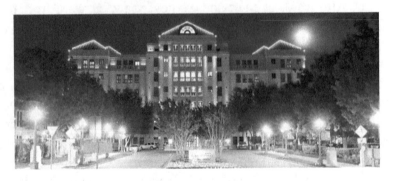

Relief

I mmediately after arriving I was rushed into the emergency room, where I was pronounced dead. When someone gets severely brain damaged or becomes brain dead, there isn't any blood flow, or oxygen to their brain. Thereby causing it and everything connected to the brain stem (the lungs) to cease function, and since I was brain dead all efforts to revive me seemed useless.

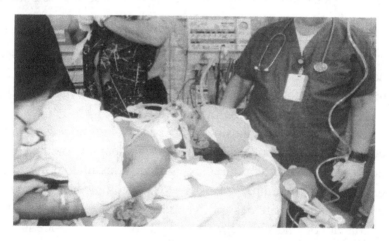

Technically speaking I still had warm blood running through my veins, canceling out the factor of death, but as long as the ventilator was breathing for me, I wasn't really living at all. After hours of waiting someone finally came out to speak to my parents.

Once the bad news arrived, my dad took it into the hall. He knew how fragile my mother was at this point, so, in an attempt to prevent her mood from worsening, he moved the conversation behind closed doors. Once outside he not only found out that I was dead, but that I would soon be transported to the morgue. After hearing these words, my dad couldn't believe it.

Never in his right mind could he imagine that such a thing would happen to me. He just couldn't believe that this was it for my life. I was just a kid who had yet to experience life to its fullest. It didn't seem fair that my life had to end so early, or that I had to die in such a way. No matter what, though, he refused to give up on me, and was determined that I would live to see another day.

Unfortunately, the doctor delivering the news disagreed. He argued back and forth with him, stating that I was dead and there was nothing more that could be done for me.

My dad missed out on being there for me prior to the wreck, and he wasn't going to let it happen again. He was determined not to leave me this time. My mother had asked if he could pick me up after school, since she was running late from her job at the F.A.A, but he chose to continue working.

He owned his own business, where he sold fragrances in and out of his vehicle, but because he chose to deny my mother's request, it lead to her not only having to pick me up, but my baby brother, too. Therefore, causing us to arrive home late, and meet with our unfortunate destiny. My dad felt guilty, so to make up for his actions he was helping to fight for my life. Once it was determined that my dad wasn't backing down, the doctor had no choice but to meet with his demands; which were to keep me on life support, and not send me to the morgue.

After their heated conversation, the doctor called everyone back on the case and prepared me for surgery. Once in place a hole was drilled into my swollen head, to release the trapped pressure. Immediately after, my head was wrapped with bandages and gauze tape. Once that was done my belly was cut open, to insert a gastrostomy tube.

Although, they thought their hard work would be in vein, the odds of making a comeback were nonexistent, but it wasn't my time to die. That night my parents contacted our immediate family, to inform them about the wreck and my condition. Once everyone found out they became devastated, but instead of worrying they came together to give support and show their love. Everyone showed up, but my grandfather was nowhere to be seen.

At that moment my grandfather was out of state, on a business trip, so that's when my grandmother gave him a call. During their conversation, my grandmother updated him about my condition. After being informed his whole mood changed. Once he heard of this, he went from being a happy business man, to a sad and concerned grandfather. It was then, as the tears rolled down his face, when he decided to come back home.

Once that decision was made, my grandfather packed his things, left his hotel, and caught a taxi to take him to the airport. After arriving, he met up with one of his coworkers. Once united, she noticed his sad behavior, so she asked if he was okay. Once asked, my grandfather confessed his troubles. After hearing about my condition, she felt his pain and knew he was sincere, because of his sad behavior and tearful eyes.

That's when she gave him a hug, assured him that everything would be okay, and that she would pray for me. Afterwards, she left his side to inform the pilot and other coworkers boarding the plane. Then once the plane became full, those coworkers told other passengers, and so on. Once the plane ascended into the sky everyone conversed about it, but my grandfather was in the dark about anyone else knowing.

Sitting front row was my grandfather looking towards the sky, as he wished for my wellbeing and health. I was very dear to his heart and he just wanted to be by side. Hours went by before the plane made it back home, so when it did my grandfather became relieved. The flight back home only lasted approximately 3 hours and 21 minutes, but for my grandfather it seemed like forever. He was so anxious to see me that he could not wait another minute.

Once the plane arrived at DFW Airport, he became relieved. He couldn't wait to get off, but first the pilot came out to speak with him. Once the pilot approached my grandfather, he apologized for his inconvenience. Afterwards he went on to say, he was sorry the wreck took place, and that I was hurt as a result. He then said that he would pray for me.

Then once the pilot spoke his peace, he returned back to his duties. Not long after, the plane doors finally opened; once that happened, a man from behind placed a hand on my grandfather's shoulder. Once he had my grandfather's attention, he let him know that everyone knew about me, and were not only praying for me to get better, but for him as well. Once that was said, my grandfather thanked the kind man and everyone involved.

Afterwards he grabbed his briefcase and departed from the plane. Once off he picked up his luggage and left the airport. Once inside his car, he drove to Cook Children's Hospital. It was very late in the night and my grandfather could not wait another minute to see me. Although he hadn't had any rest, he couldn't sleep until he knew that I was okay. As he drove through the heavy traffic, he said a prayer asking God to save my life, and to restore my health.

Once my grandfather arrived at the hospital, he met up with my grandmother. Afterwards he was taken to the top floor, where I was being held. Once there he met up with the rest of the family, where he along with everyone else wanted to see me. Unfortunately though, it could not be done. At that moment the authorities wouldn't allow anyone to see me, because I was in critical condition.

Prayer

As the night grew later into the day, my family knew they would not get a chance to see me, so they began to call family and close friends. Once in contact, all were told about my condition, and were asked to pray for me. My family knew that faith, unaccompanied by action was useless, so they also prayed. In fact hundreds of people all around, were praying for me to get better that night. This is known as the power of prayer.

The miracle prayer, if said faithfully, will bring about spiritual depth, and cause miracles to happen. These prayers spoke volumes, and that night I would soon experience the love of God, in a special way. It was very late in the night, and now it was just my parents that remained. My parents had been awake all day and their eyes grew weary and tired. They tried their best to stay awake, but there's only so much that coffee can do.

It came to the point where caffeine no longer worked and their tired minds grew restless. They just couldn't prolong their creeping eyes from closing anymore, so after praying again they rested. With all their heart they believed God would come through for them, on my behalf. Their faith was strong and they knew if it was God's will, I would make a comeback.

God responds to faith, therefore, prayer without it is nothing but dead incantation. For those that cometh to God, must believe that He is and He'll reward those that diligently seek Him. So in accordance to prayer and my family's faith, God came to my aid. It was the midnight hour, the emergency room was silent, and I was left all alone. My condition hadn't changed at all, and the authorities didn't see any improvement in my status, but it was not my time to die.

As I lay lifeless, God approached my bed side. Once in place, He spoke my name, and reached into my body. Afterwards He removed the living entity from the deceased vessel, and took me to paradise. While in His arms I stared and remained speechless. That's when He gazed back, and gave a friendly smile.

He then told me, that it wasn't my time to die, and that there was much work left to be done on earth. He also warned me that my path would not be an easy one, but help would come to those that believe in truth. Therefore, if it was truth I heard then it was coming from Him, but only those that follow His word and serve Him can ever know. During our conversation, time seemed to stand still. It seemed like we had been walking for days, until we reached a bench.

After sitting down, God began to gaze at the horizon. He then looked into my eyes and gave another smile. Next He reclined my head onto His lap, where I focused my eyes at the sky. Once that happened my mouth dropped with amazement. It was the most beautiful site I'd ever seen, and He knew I would like it.

He laughed with excitement when He saw my face light up with joy. I gazed for hours, and my mind became lost with wonder. I soon became filled with exhaustion, and began to doze off. As my eyes grew weaker, He sang to me, and pretty soon I fell asleep. The next time I awoke, was to His voice.

"It's time," He said, but I didn't know what He meant. Little did I know He was actually referring to our departure, but first He met with all the other angels. Once in place He gave my testimony, where He foretold the trials and tribulations I was to face. My hard comings, what I was to achieve, and accomplish in life. After His speech He moved towards the large group of applauding angels.

Once He approached the large crowd, three faces emerged. They were of the two angels I saw during the wreck, including the one that came to our aid afterwards. Once united, all three joined God and me as He led everyone towards a large body of standing water. Once there everyone entered the vast pool, surrounding the five of us, as we stood in the center.

Once we entered the water, every inch of my body was bathed clean; then they tilted my head back, and made me new. After being baptized I was brought back up a changed person. The boy I used to be was no more; I had a new identity and I knew my purpose. God then lifted me out of the water, and gave another speech. Once finished, He handed me over to my angel friends.

After they gave their love, He took me back to my body. Once in place, He laid my spirit back inside. Afterwards He put His healing hands over my head and heart, kissed my lips open and breathed air back into my lungs. Once that was done He kissed my forehead; after kissing my head a healing process began to take place in my brain.

Immediately after that happened I drifted to sleep, where I began to dream. Once that happened, He held my hand firmly and told me He loved me. Throughout the night, and the following morning, a miracle had taken place. The medics walked into the emergency room, expecting to see me just the way they left me, but once inside they couldn't believe what they saw. After entering the emergency room, they discovered that I was not only alive, but breathing on my own with little brain activity.

Medically speaking I should have been dead, but somehow I was resting peacefully instead. Their minds became filled with disbelief, as they tried to figure out the impossible. They just couldn't explain it, but my family knew the deal. The Devil tried to put a period to my name, but God took that period and turned it into a comma. All because He loved me, and heard my families prayers. I was now in a coma.

Imagine That

I magine living your whole life in the now, not thinking about the outcome of tomorrow. Living each day, not caring at all about what happened, what you did the day before, or the consequences you would have to pay for the foolish decisions made. Taking life for granted, and not remembering that each day lived is a gift. This was my daily life before the wreck ever happened, but what could be done about it.

It was all in my past, what's done is done, and there was nothing that I could do about that, because I was now a vegetable. As I slept, I dreamt of my stay in heaven. Each day for two and a half (2½) months, I spent another day with God. Except this time it was my mind absent from the body, instead of my spirit. On the outside I was doing remarkably well, given the circumstances.

My brain was healing every day, and my status was improving more and more. Many days went by, when my family just quietly sat and watched; all wondering what was going on in my mind. Just waiting for the day, when they could hear my voice again. For two weeks straight I laid in that bed with no sound, or movement. Then came the day when I did both.

At that time, my family was gathered around my bed side, watching as I slept. That's when I wrapped my arms around what they could not see, and spoke in a soft voice. "I love you too, you and I are one, and we are one." They knew who I was talking to, and it made them glad that I was happy with God, instead of feeling the pain written all over my face.

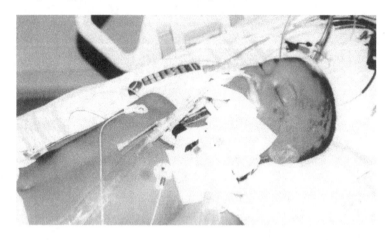

Later that week my family received a call that also made them happy.

That's when my family discovered, the woman responsible for my condition was arrested. After receiving this information, my family felt relieved. Knowing this woman was in custody, gave my family hope that justice would be served. After that call a court date was set to take place two weeks later. During that time my family was able to find and hire the best attorneys for my mother and I.

With outstanding evidence and three eye witnesses we were guaranteed to win. When the court date arrived our attorneys were sent in place of my mother and I.

The evidence we had alone was enough to put that woman away for sure, or so we thought. As the trial proceeded our attorneys fought their hardest to ensure that justice was served, but the judge showed favoritism towards the guilty. In spite of all the evidence we had stacked against her, the judge looked the other way and gave her a misdemeanor.

After all the time and hard work that was put in to find her, she was being freed back into society without probation, or even a suspended license. Who would have thought that our case would be handled in such an unjust manner? Nevertheless, once my family found out they became very upset with the judge's decision. After all, who's to say that she learned her lesson? Who's to say that she was truly sorry for what she did, and who's to say that she wouldn't do it again?

Unfortunately, my parents had absolutely no control over it. The courtroom was where the judge presided and his decision was final, so they had no choice but to let it go. Besides they still had me, and that's what mattered most. Each day for two and a half (2½) months, they watched as I slept, anticipating each day, wondering when I would awake. During this time I was also visited by many family members, close friends and relatives from in and out of state.

Day in and day out, many came to give their condolences to my family and I. Then came the day when I finally awoke out of my coma. It was on the morning of June 15, 2005. That morning, the authorities came to change my sheets. After arriving they pealed back my sheets layer by layer. That's when an unpleasant odor hit their faces.

It had been so long since I was last cleaned, and because of this my body smelled really badly. After being greeted by my stinky scent, I was taken out of my bed. Afterwards I was stripped of the diaper that I now had on, and was placed into a shower chair. After entering the open shower, the water was turned on. As the water sprinkled me, I was lathered with soap, and every inch of my body was cleaned.

Minutes into the shower, my care providers heard something. It sounded as if it was coming from me, so that's when the water was turned off. After turning off the water they found that I was not only awake, but crying too. "The water was where I was cleaned and made new, and the water is how I was reborn into the world." After awaking, I was dried off and carried back to bed, still crying.

After being laid down, I focused my attention on a figure standing in a bright light. Once in sight It spoke and said, "Jordan my son don't fright, you're safe, so be calm and rest." Its voice sounded familiar and I knew who it was, it was God. Now that I was of the living, I could no longer see His true form. Fortunately we shared a spiritual connection, and I knew it was Him.

Afterwards God placed a hand on my head, and took away all my stress and worries. Once that happened a spell fell over me, and I drifted back to sleep. For at least a month I was in a persistent vegetative state. This meant that I was in a state of partial arousal, rather than true awareness. When I opened my eyes I knew nothing of the world, I was brought back to the beginning. I was reborn with the naivety of a new born infant.

My mind had become inexperienced and just as every baby goes through developmental stages, I had to go through them all over again. However, relearning these skills was important to maintain the best quality of my life. After arousing from my stupor, I had a team of support helping restore me back to normal. During my stay at the hospital, I went through several types of therapy.

Each time strengthening different muscles in my body, but before I could do that, I needed to rebuild my back muscles. This was done by repetitiously helping me sit up straight, until I was able to do it on my own. After the restoration of my back, I began to venture outside my room, where I was wheeled around in a wheel chair.

Heaven Sent

E ach day as I ventured outside my room, I reminisced about my stay in heaven, and wondered when I would see God again. It saddened me that I couldn't be with Him, but God did not forsake me. In His place He sent angels. Running down the halls was a naked old man dressed in a hospital gown, accompanied by two nurses chasing close after. I always watched this man cause chaos, and get hounded down by the same two nurses daily.

It was hilarious and it always made me laugh. At this time I also began to notice someone in particular. She was a nurse whom I'd never seen or met before. She was very beautiful, had short curly blond hair, and always wore rose colored lipstick. I stared at this woman for days, never knowing what to say, or how to say it.

Until the day came, when I decided to try and say something. Once she heard me trying to speak to her, she replied back, said hello, and asked me how I was doing. After greeting each other, we continued conversing. Amazingly she was able to understand everything I said, even though I had no words to speak. Whenever we spent time with each other, it never dawned on me how special she was.

All that mattered was that I had a friend. No one outside of her knew that I was talking, or at least trying to. That is, until my family paid me a visit. At this time, everyone was gathered around my bedside, watching as I stared out into the open. For days I laid in that same position. It was unknown if I could talk, because other than being present, all I did was stare out into space.

For that reason alone no one knew if I could talk, but my grandfather was determined. He had waited months to hear my voice again, and he wasn't going to let another day pass him by. That's when he asked me if I could say Papa. With great expectation everyone was waiting to hear if I could say it, or not. For a minute there was an awkward silence, until everyone saw my lips move very slowly to say, Papa."

Although my grandfather saw it with his own eyes, he still couldn't believe I said it. That's when my grandfather confronted my dad to stop, as he often times would mess around with my grandfather. He could swear that was my dad's voice he heard, but when my dad said it wasn't him, my grandfather just asked me to say papa again, and as I did before, I said it once more. Everyone became filled with joy, and my grandfather was so happy, that he became full of smiles.

As the time grew later into the day, I became filled with fatigue and fell asleep. I awoke the next morning with posing questions that I've had for quite some time. Where is my nurse friend, I usually spoke with her daily, but for some reason hadn't seen her or that crazy old man? That is, until they both paid me a visit. Once inside my room they both greeted me with smiles.

That's when my nurse friend congratulated me on my success. Afterwards she told me how proud of me she was, and then went on to say that she knew I could do it. Afterwards she told me how much she was going to miss me, and that she loved me. That's when she revealed, that she and the old man were guardian angels sent by God to watch over me.

After revealing their secret, she told me that I would no longer be able to see them, but not to worry because we would meet each other again someday. After her speech they both gave me hugs, then they left. When God sends His angels it's to rescue, guard, keep, & protect in all ways to carry out his desires, each case is different and in my mind they were sent with a purpose.

Each time I saw that crazy old man it made me laugh, and feel better about myself. Whenever I conversed with my nurse friend, it was rebuilding my vocal muscles. She also served as my friend, which helped me to realize that I wasn't alone. She helped me see that God, herself, and all my family, were behind me every step of the way. She helped me realize that the following people would be with me until the very end.

All of these people were responsible for my progression. Each person played a part in my healing and now the rest was left up to me, as I continued down the long road to recovery.

Recovery

After the departure of my friends, I was no longer unsure of my ability to talk. I embraced my weak voice, and spoke freely. Once word spread that I was trying to talk, I began participating in speech therapy. During that time I relearned vocabulary and strengthened my voice, later being able to form words, full sentences, and hold brief conversations. It was also at this point when my family discovered a change in my behavior.

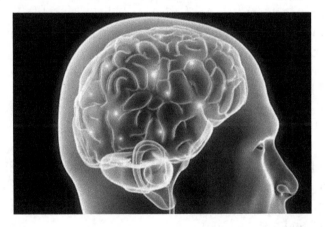

The brain heals in mysterious ways, and I was now very sensitive to noise, as well as having emotional liability. This meant that I was happy one moment, sad the next, and angry another. This was not the Jordan my family remembered. It also struck a lot of questions, as to why I was acting in such a way. These mood swings that I was experiencing were caused by damage to my cerebrum. This particular part of the brain controls emotions and behavior, which explained mine. However, my family did not abandon me. No matter how bad my mental state became, my family never left my side.

Instead they worked with me, helping me to see this wasn't the proper way to act. Another thing my injury caused was problems with cognition. This made it hard to remember current events and information I normally knew, or would have been able to recall. Such as, from something that happened only seconds or minutes ago, to a memorable event that happened in my past. Many times I would forget where I was, faces I saw on a daily basis, and voices I heard in the past.

The one thing I did seem to remember was a question in my mind. A recurring question, I could never remember long enough to ask. That is until a bright light peered down towards me, and out of this light appeared a man. He spoke to me and I was not frightened, because His voice sounded familiar. In His presence I was finally able to verbalize my thoughts, but first I asked for His name.

Once, asked He replied back and said His name was Jesus. After learning His name, I asked the same question I kept asking myself. "Why am I here?" An answer that I'm sure was revealed to me in the past, but I didn't have any memory to recall. Once asked, Jesus told me that I was in a wreck, but that there was no need to worry, because I was safe. Afterwards He told me to be calmed and rest.

Once that was said a spell fell over me, and as my eyes crept closed, Jesus placed a hand over my confused head, and relieved me of all my stress and worries. Once that was done He left me to sleep. The next time I awoke, I no longer wondered why I was in a hospital. I was now able to remember where I was, and why

I was there. Therefore, on Jesus' previous visit, He gave me a gift. He gave me a piece of my memory back, and the ability to remember.

Once this change occurred I was able to remember things, as they happened in my present, allowing me to become more productive and cooperative whenever my doctors, nurses, therapist, or family walked into my room. I now understood my circumstances, and knew that they were only there to help me. Once my behavior returned to normal I was enrolled into hospital school, where I relearned basic education and regained academic progress.

In class I not only relearned forgotten material, but experienced what it was like to work with other disabled kids, eventually helping me to become comfortable with my circumstances, going to school and working alongside others. Outside of school I went through several types of therapy, where I continuously exercised my weak, unused muscles. Many days passed when I wanted to quit, but I kept going because I had motivation.

Motivation

During my stay at Cook Children's Hospital, I received visits on numerous occasions. These visits consisted of many different people. Most of the time it was family, other times it was a story teller, a clown, or a gift bearer. Each time it was someone new, taking the time out of their day to make me happy. Whenever these people visited it was to provide company, entertain, or give their love in all ways to make me feel better and uplift my spirit.

I witnessed the happiness they created in other patients, and admired the way they made me feel. In fact this would depict my career choice later in life, but for the time being, I enjoyed the moment while it lasted. Not long after receiving this motivation, I began believing in myself, and became self-confident. I could do anything if I just put my mind to it. Nothing was unachievable; all things were in my reach.

I was given a second chance at life for a reason, and I wasn't going to let it go to waste. I soon began to understand that nothing in life would ever come easily, and if I wanted to achieve my goals, I would have to work my hardest to do so. Quitting was not an option, because I now had the tenacity to keep going.

Once this happened my progress in therapy improved. Not only were my muscles growing stronger, but I also began to walk. I was moving mountains, with the faith of a mustard seed. I was doing what was said could not be done, based in the belief that I could do, or be anything if I put my mind to it. Sure my ability to do some things perfectly was no longer there; at least I still had a life to live.

As long as that factor was in effect, new talents could be developed and take the place of what was lost. Therefore, each day lived not only brought with it purpose, but new opportunities as well. Knowing this information gave me strength to continue moving forward. This new sense of hope taught me not to give up, and to never stop trying. Once I realized my full potential, not only did my walking improve, but so did my participation in therapy.

Once that occurred I was released from the hospital, but God wasn't finished with me yet. Over the following months, and next couple of years my time would be spent in therapy, so that I could continue strengthening my muscles, but first came the weekend. It was a Friday night and I was so exhausted that after arriving home I crashed into my bed and rested.

The next day was spent with my family, where I learned more about my past, and saw a glimpse of what used to be. I spent hours, flipping through portfolio pages and looking at old frames. I also saw many awards, representing all the achievements that I'd made in the past. All these items told a story about a chapter from my life I no longer remembered. Through these pictures I saw the same smiling face over, and over again.

It was me, but at the same time it wasn't. I was no longer the same person, I used to be. It was like seeing a stranger, as I looked through these items I wondered who this person was, what his inner thoughts were like, and tried to draw some kind of correlation between who I used to be and who I was now, but could not relate. These things no longer mattered to me.

I felt my purpose in life was greater, and that surviving my trials and tribulations defined who I am. My passion for life was no longer for myself, but for God and others in need. I now had the desire to tell my story, so that others could experience the love of God too. From that moment on I decided to live my life differently. No longer would I think of myself, nor do selfish deeds. Instead I would think of others, and do for them what was done for me.

I would become a positive force in the eyes of God, myself and others. This was my second chance at life, and this time I would live life the way it was intended to be. For the moment, though I slept. Therefore, it was the night of, and tomorrow would mark the beginning of, a new chapter.

Turning Point

The next day I was awakened by my mother. It was Sunday morning and the delicious aroma of food filled the air. Once out of bed, I joined my family to have breakfast. Once my stomach was filled, I left to get cleaned up. Afterwards I returned to my room, to discover ironed dress cloths laid out, for me to wear.

After dressing myself, I walked out my room to find my family all dressed and waiting. That's when we went out to the family car, then after strapping in we headed down the road to Great Commission Baptist Church.

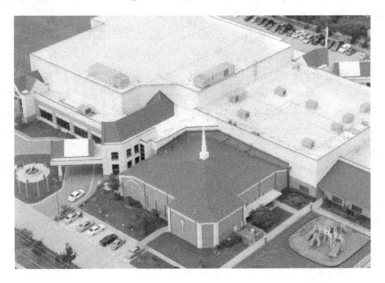

Once we arrived I didn't know what to think. I had no idea what we were doing there, or what was about to take place. After departing from our car, we walked towards the church. Once inside, we were greeted by an usher at the door. Once greeted, my dad left us to speak to another usher inside the sanctuary.

That usher went to tell the pastor that I was there. Once Pastor Brown found out, he informed my grandfather. Then, after receiving this news my grandfather took over on the microphone. Once in place he informed the audience about the wreck, explained that I wasn't expected to see another day, and then he became so full of the Spirit that he just told me to "come on in."

As I entered the sanctuary the whole church began to cheer and applaud. Inside I felt God's presence all around, although I couldn't see Him I knew He was with me. After approaching the stage, I was helped up the small stair way to the podium. Once in place, I thanked everyone for their prayers, at the same time trying to think of what to say next. There was so much I wanted to say, but didn't know how to put it to words, until I felt God's touch, encouraging me to keep going.

At that moment, I began to remember all the things He brought me through. How I survived the wreck, how I was able to recoup from my injuries, and how I was able to make it out of the hospital. Through it all, God never left my side. He was with me every step of the way, and because of it there I stood, not only a living, breathing, and functioning being, but a testament to His glory.

Immediately after this happened, I began to shout hallelujah and once that happened I couldn't contain myself. I was filled with the Holy Spirit, and my praise became continuous. Once that happened I couldn't control myself. What was intended to be a warming for my arrival quickly became a celebration for life, and my exuberance was so contagious, that the whole church joined me in praise.

Once everyone settled down, Pastor Brown preached one heck of a sermon. When church ended I was taken back home with a new lease on life. Right after my moment on stage, I began to feel different. All of a sudden, I felt as if that single moment defined who I am. I felt that my calling in life was to give testament to the blind and give hope to the hopeless.

From that moment on I decided to live life differently. No longer would I selfishly think of, or do for myself. Instead I would do for others, what was done for me. I would give motivation to those in need, and spread positivity everywhere I went. I would become a positive force in the eyes of myself, and others.

I would also do the best of my ability to be a good person, and lead by example. I would do all that I could to ensure success, and become a good man. I felt it was my destiny, and knew that with God on my side all these things were possible. By the end of that day my mind was made and I knew what I was to become; a motivational speaker.

In my heart I felt I was making the right decision, but I needed to be sure. That's when I asked God for His guidance, and it was during that day when He provided an answer. Later that night as I slept, I dreamt. In this precognitive dream, I was an adult standing behind a podium. At that moment one word escaped my mouth, "Thank you;" afterwards the audience, below applauded and cheered.

That's when a beautiful woman carrying a baby rushed onto stage, congratulated me, wrapped her arm around me, and kissed my lips. I kissed her back and couldn't stop from smiling. I then turned forward, where I saw a bright figure standing amongst the applauding crowd. It was God, and as I made an attempt to wave at Him I awoke to my mother. After awaking from my dream I knew what was to come, and that I was making the right decision with my career choice.

From that day out I would work my hardest at becoming the best motivational speaker I could be, but first I needed an education. It was now Monday morning, and I would soon begin my first day back in school.

School

O nce I returned to school all my teachers and friends were really excited to see me. The last time any of them did was on a fieldtrip to Cook Children's Hospital. Everyone knew my situation, and it made them glad that I was well and present. As the morning progressed I was certain my first day back in school would be great, but I spoke to soon.

I thought my first day back would be like hospital school, but soon found out differently. As my day progressed I discovered that, I could no longer keep up with my class mates, or comprehend what was being taught. Not only could I not understand the material being given, but I had no idea how to do it. Although I gave my best effort, the work was just way too advanced for my mind to grasp. I needed help, help that this school could no longer provide.

Unfortunately, that wasn't my only problem. Later that day I discovered that my friends resented me. Many of them remembered who I was before the wreck, and just couldn't except that I was different now. Some turned their noses when I couldn't meet their expectations. It didn't matter how good of a person I was in the past. What mattered most was that I wasn't cool enough to hang with them anymore.

My friends wanted the old Jordan back, instead of accepting the new, and improved version. There was no doubt that my friends didn't like these new changes and I was getting ready to find out just, how much one person really disliked them. After school I was pulled aside, by someone I once called my girl-friend. During that time she told me she couldn't be my friend anymore, because I was retarded.

Once that was said, she started making fun of me in front of our friends. I was hurt over the fact that she could even do something like that, but what hurt me most was the look on my friends face afterwards. Not a single one of them stood up for me, or said anything in my defense. Instead they each stood with their heads down, looking sorry. Did they agree? I didn't stick around long enough to find out. I felt angry, sad, humiliated and betrayed.

I just couldn't believe that these were the same people that cried, after hearing about the wreck. I couldn't believe these were the same people that felt compassion and sympathy for me, when I was sick. The one thing I was sure about is that I no longer had friends. I just didn't understand why being so differ-ent was such a bad thing, nor did I understand why I was being mistreated. Was it my fault?

No matter what I did, though, I just couldn't make any since of it. Once my mother came to pick me up I told her all about my bad day, including the altercation between my friends and I. I also told her how much I hated school, and that I didn't want to go back. Once this was said, my mother expressed her sym-pathy for my pain and misfortune. She was sorry that I had to go through that, but explained to me how some people are quick to judge from what they see on the outside, instead of getting to know that person for who they are.

As for the miseducation I received throughout my classes, I wouldn't have to worry about that anymore. Once I told my mother about my troubles, she knew it was time for a change. So that day she pulled me out of my school and started looking for others that would cope with my disabilities. The search for the right school was a very difficult process. Each school had its own defining characteristic, that made it a valuable pick, but it needed to be right.

With patience and help from God a decision was finally made, on a school named Jackie Carden. This school was just like any other, but what set it apart was one teacher named Mrs. Jenesta. This teacher was different from all the rest, because she also had a brain injury. She knew all about what I was going though, because she went through it herself. Once I started going to this school I no longer felt alone about my condition, because I had someone to share it with.

Continuing Education

During my 5th grade year learning was a challenge. There was little that I knew for my grade level and my memory loss prevented me from retaining new information. For those reasons I was placed into special education, so that I could achieve a higher level of self-sufficiency and success. With the combination of help from my teachers and certified accommodations, I was able to make it. Therefore, these changes were necessary for me to succeed.

Without the needed accommodations, I wouldn't have been able to make it through school. With that being said my 5th grade year was a success. Once I completed the 5th grade, I joined a school in Burleson named Hughes Middle School. Once enrolled, I was placed back into Special Ed. As a bonus I would also receive both physical therapy and occupational therapy once a month, as well as Adaptive P.E.

At this school all my teachers loved me, and made it their job to make sure I never got left behind, and I passed all my classes. For three, long years I worked to the best of my ability, until I made it out of the 8th grade. Once school ended, I enjoyed a much needed summer. Once summer was over, I began my first year of high school. During my freshmen year I continued to receive therapy, as well as adaptive P.E, and Special Ed. services throughout all my classes.

High school was a new scene for me. It was ferocious in size, and it was very easy for me to get lost and confused, but I was able to make it with help. Once I started school, I was enrolled into the PASS Program. Within this program I had three different teachers. Each did their share with helping me throughout school. With their help I was able to resolve conflicts, and learn my way throughout the building.

With the help of this program and my Special Education classes, I was able to make it throughout my 9th and 10th grade year. I was achieving success and seemed to be happy, but I wasn't. Each day spent at school was extremely difficult for me; the work was very hard and confusing. Many times I was also mistreated by my peers, and felt like an outcast. I felt like I was unwanted and disliked in every way.

It seemed like the abuse would never stop, and because of it I started hating myself. I began to believe what everyone said about me was true, and wished that I was dead. I was slowly deteriorating from within. My humanity was being wiped out, and my unique qualities were taken over by a negative entity. I was on the verge of destruction, and wanted to give up.

I was defeated and began to feel less of a man. I was lost without any hope, and didn't know what to do. That's when I decided to take back control of my life. I was tired of living in doubt and fear, and I realized that I was more than what my limitations allowed me to be. I was not going to let my disabilities get in the way of living my life, and I refused to give up. Once I realized my full potential, I became unstoppable.

I was conquering all barriers standing in my way. Nothing could stop me now. I was on a mission to achieve success, and my light shined so brightly that others took attention to it. One person in particular was Steve Harvey. At the beginning of my junior year I entered an essay contest for Mr. Harvey and Essence Magazine, and it wasn't until this change occurred when I received a reply back.

Once that day came, I discovered that I was one out of one hundred students in the United States chosen to go to Disney World, and partake in an event called Dreamers Academy.

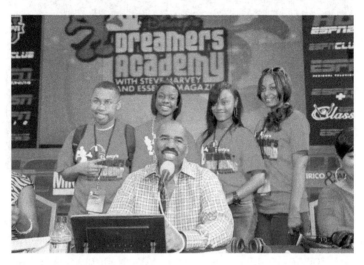

During my stay in Disney World I learned the importance of self and dreaming big. I also made many friends, and met allot of people. Among those people were Ruben Studard, Kimberly Lock, Yolanda Adams, Tia Mowry, Terence J, Raven Symoné, and Mr. Harvey himself. My time in Disney World lasted for 3½ days, and on the fourth day, I received an award for my outstanding dream to become a motivational speaker. Afterwards I graduated from the academy, and went back home.

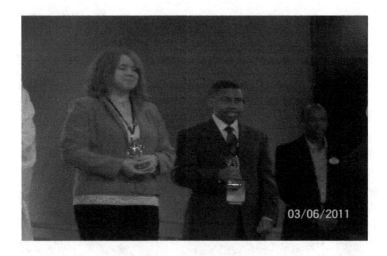

03/06/2011

Dreamers Academy was a life changer for me. It was a sign that my living had not been in vein, and that I was on the right path to success. Although my stay was short lived, I wouldn't trade it for anything in the world. My experience was one that many dreamed of, and I didn't take that for granted. I was going to use what I learned to benefit my life, and help construct my future.

Now all that remained was the completion of my junior year. Therefore, the next day began my first week back in school. Once that day arrived, I returned to school with a new lease on life. My experience from the academy helped me realize my full potential, and because of it I knew that continuing my education was the key to achieving my goals.

Even if my journey to success took forever to accomplish, I wasn't going to give up. I had confidence in myself and knew if I put my mind to it, anything was possible. As long as I had hope, no giant was too big to conquer. I was on a mission to achieve greatness, and I wasn't going to stop until I was success-ful. Once I returned to school, I was ready.

I wasn't afraid of anything, whatever school threw at me I could take it. I've come too far to stop now I kept telling myself, and in no time at all I successfully passed another school year. Soon after school ended, I enjoyed another summer. During that time I had plenty of fun, time to kick back and relaxed. In fact, I had so much fun that time seemed to fly by, and before I knew it I was in school once more for my for my long anticipated senior year.

Senior Year

I had finally made it to 2012, my last and final year of High School, where I was welcomed back into the school with open arms. There the work was very different from last years', but with hard work, dedication and help from my peers I was able to make it throughout the year. Once again I was assisted by my teachers where they taught me how to do the new curriculum at hand.

Each and every day was filled with studies where I was learning things that would, hopefully, benefit me later in life. Whenever those studies were finished I took a test, one after the other in each subject. Just to prepare me for another test down the road. Exams that would decipher whether or not I would move on to the next chapter in my education and life.

But I would be lying if I said doing work and taking tests was all that I did. My days were also filled with senior skip days, picnics, tail gate parties, and lastly, prom and project celebration. In the midst of all this and as the days starting counting down to graduation, I decided to submit an application online to Howard County College, where I would later attend school.

For weeks I waited for a reply back, and at the same time I was also going to school trying to finish out the rest of the year there. So after a couple of weeks I finally received a reply back from the college, stating that they received my application and that I had been accepted into the school. Now all that was left to do was take my final exams. When the time finally came to take those exams I was so exhausted from the many days of school that I was actually glad that I could finally take them, so that I could go ahead and knock them out the way and move on.

I tried my best on every single one of them, although I did struggle on at least two. I knew that I would come out victorious. Because I'd come too far to let some test that says nothing about my character or the type of person I am stop me from achieving success and fulfilling my destiny. So I took each day as it came by slowly. I accomplished this by remaining calm and staying focused, until I took all of my exams.

I was finally finished, I had completed all of my final exams and now summer was just a day away. I've always loved summer, so you know when it came I had no problem with letting loose and having fun. Early that summer I also started getting ready for graduation: the highlight of that year, the final chapter of my boyhood, and the first step into manhood. By this time I was so anxious to walk that stage and receive my high school diploma that I could barely wait.

When graduation finally came on June 5th of that year I became so excited because I could now get my high school diploma and get on with my life. Graduation took place in a lobby on the inside of a hotel, and during this time many special awards were given out for one reason or another, and although I did not receive any for my achievements in life, I was not upset; because I've already accomplished so much more than anyone there could ever know.

I'm not lucky, I'm blessed to be alive and to have journeyed this far, but my life won't end here. I will continue to grow, and move forward. I've come too far to stop now. I will continue striving forward achieving anything and everything I put my mind to and to think those seven years ago I could have been dead, but look at me now. I'm successful; I'm achieving my dreams and living my life to the fullest.

I refuse to let my disabilities get in the way of living my life, and I won't let a near death experience scar me. I've come too far to stop now. I will keep striving forward achieving anything and everything I put my mind to. Only good things can come from this and the best has yet to come, I know this because I walk by faith. Faith is what brought me this far, hope is what keeps me looking forward, and determination is what keeps me going. I will believe in self and trust in God all the way because I know that through him all things are possible.

I will continue achieving my dreams and living life to the fullest. I won't let my disabilities get in the way, and I won't let a near death experience scar me. So will I ever give up? No I won't! I refuse; the choice to live life is mine and I choose to live it. To give up would be abuse not only to me but to God as well and anybody else that thinks their life is a living hell. So my advice to you the reader is to hang in there a little longer. You didn't get to where you are now by some dumb four leaf clover.

Luck had nothing to do with this. You have a purpose in life too. Hope, faith, belief in self and God got me where I am today, so try it for yourself and see where it gets you. This is not a fictional story; therefore, it contains nothing but facts. This is not a story of triumph, but instead it's one of success. This is a story of life, my life.

One of truth and inside these truths contains the steps I took to become the person I am today. So read it closely, and apply it to life and I hope that it will help you throughout yours.

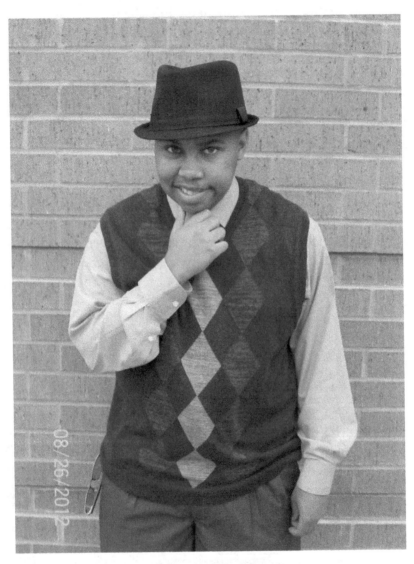

The End

The Conclusion

God never puts more on us then we can handle. Therefore, our experiences in life occur for a reason, and that reason is to ensure success. Although these incidents may seem like a curse, it's actually a blessing in disguise. Therefore, without trial and error we wouldn't make mistakes, without mistakes we wouldn't know the difference between right and wrong, and without the obtained knowledge we wouldn't be successful.

As for my life, the wreck was tragic and what happened to me was unfortunate, but in order for God to reach my heart it had to be done. God never intended for me to get hurt or die. The very fact that that ordeal happened, was just another example of the devil trying to rob me of my destiny. Fortunately God kept a watchful eye over me. He saved my life and allowed me to live through it, enabling me to gain wisdom throughout my experience and change my fate.

I thank God every day for my second chance at life and past experiences, because without the benefitting factors from them, where would I be? Before the wreck happened, I was an ordinary person with ordinary dreams. I was living a negative life style and could care less about where I was headed, or what happened to me along the way. I only cared about myself and was willing to do anything to reach my goals. Unfortunately the plans I had for myself didn't line up with the ones God had in store for my life.

God saw something in me that I didn't see in myself, but I was hard headed and ignored all the signs given. So in order to get through to me He allowed the wreck to happen. I was in His hands the whole time and what seemed to be the end, was actually a new beginning for my life. Therefore, in order to truly hear what He was saying, death had to occur. That way I was not only listening with my mind, but my soul as well.

His words were deeply ingrained into my heart, and became the muscle that kept it beating. Once that happened my life changed for the better. He opened my eyes to all the possibilities available for me. He shifted my attention away from the world's influence, and made me realize that all my past aspirations weren't for me. He showed me my full potential, and helped me realize my true calling in life.

My dream is to motivate and inspire. I hope to make a difference in the lives of many, by telling my story. I want give hope and strength to all that hear my voice, and I want to inspire many to strive forward and achieve success for their lives. My testimony is one of triumph; one I hope will help many to overcome whatever they're going through. We're only human, but if we have hope, put faith in God and ourselves we can do anything.

With that in mind all things are possible. I know this because I'm a living witness of what God can do and if He did it for me; I just know He can do it for you too. I am Jordan Murrell "The Motivational Speaker."

CPSIA information can be obtained
at www.ICGtesting.com
Printed in the USA
JSHW030815170222
22907JS00005B/146